# EAT SLEEP AND TRAIN

## FAT LOSS AND MUSCLE GAIN

### SMART STRATEGIES FOR YOUR GYM TIME

DIVA SELAH JOANNA

© Diva Selah Joanna 2024

Ebook ISBN 978-1-7636520-0-2

Paperback ISBN 978-1-7636520-3-3

Hardcover ISBN 978-1-7636520-2-6

**Content Warning and Disclaimer:**

This book contains discussions of mental health issues, including depression, anxiety, and personal struggles. Some chapters may include descriptions of distressing experiences and emotional challenges that might be triggering to some readers. Reader discretion is advised.

The author of this book is not a licensed nutritionist or professional health trainer. The information provided is based on personal experiences and research and is for educational and motivational purposes only and should not replace professional medical advice or treatment. Readers should consult with a qualified healthcare professional before making any significant changes to their diet or exercise routine. The author disclaims any loss, claim or damage arising from the use or misuse of the suggestions and information presented in this book.

Cover Image: Bojan, PixelStudio

Internal Layout Design: Dawn Black

# CONTENTS

# INTRODUCTION

As I cradled my newborn son in my arms, caressing his tiny fingers and delicate features, I couldn't help but be struck by the profound simplicity of his existence. For him, the world revolved around three basic necessities: food, sleep and play. In his eyes, these were not mundane tasks but essential components of his growth, development and happiness.

As a first-time mother, I embarked on a journey of discovery alongside my son, navigating the intricacies of parenthood while learning invaluable lessons about the fundamental elements of life. It was a journey marked by countless sleepless nights, messy mealtimes and joyous milestones as my son gradually mastered the art of eating, sleeping and playing.

In witnessing my son's journey from infancy to toddlerhood, I was struck by the realisation that these seemingly simple tasks were anything but trivial. They were the building blocks upon which his physical health, cognitive development and emotional well-being were constructed. Yet, as adults, we often take these basic necessities for granted, forgetting the profound significance they hold in shaping our lives.

This book is dedicated to my son, who taught me to appreciate the beauty and importance of life's simplest pleasures. It all began when he was born during the summer of January 2022. It is also a reflection on my own journey, marked by struggles with weight, body image and the profound impact that mastering the balance of eating, sleeping and training has had on my physical and mental health which eventually led me to make the most courageous decision to start my journey of motherhood as a single parent.

Through personal anecdotes, practical tips and insights derived from both my personal research and lived experience, I invite you to join me on a journey of rediscovery. Though I am not a health and nutrition expert, I offer these reflections with humility and honesty, sharing the lessons I have learned through trial and error and the wisdom I have gained along the way. Together, let us explore the transformative power of embracing the fundamentals of health and happiness: nourishing our bodies with wholesome food, prioritising rest and rejuvenation and finding joy and fulfilment in training our bodies.

As we begin this journey together, may we be inspired to reclaim our innate connection to the rhythms of life. Let us embrace the simple yet profound truth that by mastering the secrets of eating, sleeping, training and discovering their balance that suits each body, we unlock the key to a life filled with vibrant health, boundless energy and lasting happiness.

# PART ONE

# SLEEP

# CHAPTER 1:

# THE IMPORTANCE OF SLEEP

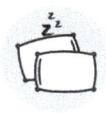

My realisation of the intricate world of sleep began with the birth of my son, a tiny bundle of joy whose arrival heralded a whirlwind of emotions and experiences unlike any I had ever felt. As a single mother, navigating the tumultuous waters of parenthood alone, I found myself grappling with the daunting task of ensuring my son's well-being, particularly when it came to the elusive art of sleep during the entirety of his first year.

The first four months of my son's life were marked by extreme sleepless nights and endless cries that kept even the neighbours awake, as he struggled with colic and discomfort that seemed to defy all attempts at comfort and consolation. Desperate for relief and guidance, I enrolled us for a week at a welcoming family care centre, where compassionate nurses and caregivers provided invaluable insights into the mysteries of infant sleep.

The first night at the centre was nothing short of a trial by fire. It took four nurses and a full two hours to finally settle my baby to sleep. As they worked tirelessly, one nurse remarked, "*This is one determined baby*", while another noted, "*Your baby's lungs are very strong*". Their comments were a mix of empathy and humour, but I was beyond exhausted. Amidst this chaotic symphony, an elderly nurse handed me a pair of earplugs, offering a gentle smile, "*Just in case*", she said, understandingly, as the cries of my baby seemed to reverberate like the combined roar of a million atomic bombs.

It was here that I learned the importance of creating a conducive sleep environment for my son. This included a pitch-black room without a hint of light, swaddling him snugly in a comforting wrap with his arms positioned above his head and softly playing gentle melodies in the background to soothe his restless mind. By embracing these simple yet profound practices, I discovered a newfound sense of calm and serenity as my son drifted off into peaceful sleep by the fourth night.

As I witnessed my son surrender to peaceful sleep, I was struck by the profound realisation that sleep is not just a state of rest, but a vital foundation of health and well-being. The absence of quality sleep can leave us feeling agitated and disconnected from ourselves. Surprisingly, it takes an entire first year of our lives to truly master the art of sleep! A whole year! Reflecting on my journey through motherhood, I realised that the most challenging aspect of the first year was establishing healthy sleep habits for my son. From needing six naps a day as an infant to just two by his first birthday, it was a gradual process that grew easier with each passing day.

Infants learn to sleep by seamlessly linking sleep cycles, paving the way for peaceful, uninterrupted nights. During sleep, the body initiates its miraculous processes of growth and repair, with each breath and heartbeat nurturing the seeds of life within. For newborns, sleep signifies a period of unparalleled growth and transformation, where their tiny bodies undergo miraculous changes in the quiet of the night. Indeed, when a newborn sleeps, they aren't simply resting; they are actively participating in the sacred task of building and growing their bodies.

And yet, the significance of sleep goes beyond infancy, impacting every aspect of human life. As adults, we also rely on sleep as a crucial component of health and vitality, a time when the body's intricate systems are given the opportunity to repair, replenish and rejuvenate.

In my own life, I have experienced firsthand the transformative power of sleep, particularly in relation to my fitness journey. As a regular at the gym, I have noticed that the days when I push myself the hardest during my workouts are usually the same days when I experience the most profound and restorative sleep.

This phenomenon can be understood through the intricate relationship between exercise and sleep, as the body's muscles undergo repair and growth during periods of rest. Intense exercise, like strength training, leads to microscopic tears and trauma in muscle fibres, prompting the body to commence repair and regeneration during sleep. Within these precious hours of slumber, the body's miraculous processes of muscle growth and repair unfold, as cells diligently mend the tears caused by training, thus enhancing physical strength and resilience. And so, it is no wonder that those who prioritise exercise often experience the reward of deep and rejuvenating sleep, as their bodies work in harmony to nurture and sustain the temple of their being.

# CHAPTER 2:

# THE TRANSFORMATIVE POWER OF SLEEP

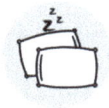

Sleep is essential for health and well-being, as it is a vital process that sustains and rejuvenates every aspect of our being. From the tangible realms of the body to the intangible realms of the mind, heart and soul, the benefits of sleep extend far beyond mere rest and relaxation. Sleep involves a comprehensive blend of physical, mental, emotional and spiritual renewal.

At its most basic level, sleep is essential for maintaining optimal physical health and vitality. It is during sleep that the body engages in a myriad of essential processes, such as repairing damaged tissues, synthesising essential hormones to bolster the immune system and regulating metabolic function. Adequate sleep is essential for promoting overall longevity, resilience and vitality, serving a crucial role in achieving optimal physical well-being.

Quality sleep also contributes to cognitive function, memory consolidation and emotional regulation. It is during sleep that the brain processes and integrates the myriad of stimuli and experiences encountered throughout the day, weaving them into the fabric of our consciousness and shaping our perceptions of the world. Adequate sleep is essential for maintaining mental clarity, focus and productivity, while chronic sleep deprivation has been linked to cognitive deficits, mood disturbances and can lead to an increased risk of mental health disorders.

Throughout history, dreams during sleep have been revered as a sacred conduit for divine guidance, creative inspiration and spiritual revelation. It is during sleep that our subconscious mind communicates with us through symbols, archetypes and metaphors, offering glimpses into the deeper truths of our existence and the mysteries of the universe. In the silent sanctuary of sleep, we are granted access to the infinite wisdom that resides within us, tapping into a wellspring of creativity, intuition and inner guidance that transcends the boundaries of the conscious mind.

In my personal journey, I have come to understand the impact of sleep on my fitness endeavours. The nights following my most intense workouts often lead to deeply restorative slumbers, during which my body replenishes and rejuvenates itself, preparing me for the challenges of the next day. Conversely, I have witnessed how a night of restless sleep can cast a pall over the following day, leaving me feeling drained and devoid of the energy needed to tackle my training. It's a cyclical dance where the quality of my sleep directly influences my ability to perform in the gym and vice versa. When sleep suffers, so does my motivation and drive to train, creating a challenging cycle to break. It serves as a reminder of the integral role that sleep plays in our overall well-being, shaping not only our physical health but also our mental resilience and motivation to pursue our fitness goals.

# Tips on how to have better sleep

Adults need somewhere between 7 and 9 hours of sleep per night. For many of us, achieving a restful night's sleep can feel like an elusive dream, as we toss and turn amidst the tangled sheets of insomnia and restlessness. Below are some tips for a good night's sleep[1].

*Exercise Regularly*: A lack of sleep can reduce your quality of life in many ways and is associated with poor physical and mental performance. One of the most well-established methods to promote healthy sleep is to engage in regular exercise. Exercise may help you feel physically tired at night, making it easier to fall asleep and promoting a more restful sleep. It may also help you unwind mentally, improve stress management and reduce anxiety.

*Create a Sleep-Inducing Environment:* Transform your bedroom into a tranquil oasis of relaxation by minimising noise, light and distractions. Invest in blackout curtains to block out unwanted light, use earplugs or white noise machines to drown out noise pollution and keep electronic devices out of reach to minimise distractions and promote a sense of calm and serenity.

**Establish a Consistent Sleep Schedule:** Set a regular bedtime and wake-up time and stick to it, even on weekends. By establishing a consistent sleep-wake cycle, you can regulate your body's internal clock, making it easier to fall asleep and wake up feeling refreshed and rejuvenated.

**Practice Relaxation Techniques:** Incorporate relaxation techniques such as deep breathing, progressive muscle relaxation, or meditation into your bedtime routine to help calm the mind and prepare your body for sleep. Engage in calming activities such as reading a book, taking a warm bath, or practising gentle yoga to signal to your body that it's time to wind down and relax.

**Limit Stimulants and Electronics Before Bed:** It is advisable to avoid engaging in stimulating activities and consuming substances such as caffeine, nicotine and alcohol in the hours before bedtime. These substances can disrupt sleep patterns and interfere with your ability to fall asleep. Similarly, minimise exposure to electronic devices such as smartphones, tablets and computers, as the blue light emitted by these devices can suppress the production of melatonin, a hormone that regulates sleep-wake cycles.

**Maintain a Comfortable Sleep Environment:** Invest in a comfortable mattress and supportive pillows that provide adequate support for your body and promote proper spinal alignment. Keep your bedroom cool, quiet and well-ventilated. Consider using a humidifier or air purifier to create an optimal sleep environment. Experiment with different sleep surfaces and bedding materials to find what works best for you, whether it's a firm mattress, soft pillows, or breathable cotton sheets.

**Limit Daytime Naps:** While daytime napping can be tempting, especially when you're feeling tired or fatigued, it can disrupt your sleep-wake cycle and make it harder to fall asleep at night. If you must nap during the day, limit it to 20-30 minutes and avoid napping late in the afternoon or evening.

**Manage Stress and Anxiety:** Practice stress management techniques such as mindfulness meditation, journaling, or engaging in hobbies and activities that bring you joy and relaxation. Seek support from friends, family, or a mental health professional if you are struggling with stress, anxiety, or other emotional issues that may be impacting your sleep.

***Consult a Healthcare Professional:*** If you continue to have trouble sleeping despite trying these tips, consider seeking advice from a healthcare professional. They can help identify underlying medical conditions or sleep disorders that may be contributing to your sleep difficulties and provide personalised recommendations and treatment options to help you achieve a restful night's sleep.

As my son reached his first birthday, an extraordinary transformation occurred, replacing the turbulent nights of infancy with a newfound sense of peace and tranquillity. No longer were the nights filled with restless cries and weary sighs; instead, sleep became a gentle companion, gracing us with its presence for a full 11 hours each night.

*Every night, as the clock struck 7:30 p.m., a familiar ritual unfolded. As his eyelids grew heavy with sleep and a wide yawn hinted that bedtime was near, I dressed him in cosy pyjamas, wrapping him in the comfort of soft cotton and warm embraces. Then, we offered a playful prayer of gratitude, giving thanks for the day's blessings and seeking protection through the night. Finally, he listened to some bedtime stories about ice cream trucks and owl hoots until he drifted off to a soothing sleep.*

In this nightly ritual, I am reminded of sleep as a gift — a gift as precious as the air we breathe and the water we drink. Just as our mobile phones require a battery charge to function properly, our bodies also require rest to repair and restore. In the quiet hours of the night, as we surrender to the gentle embrace of sleep, our bodies engage in a miraculous process of renewal, repairing the wear and tear of the day and preparing us for the challenges that lie ahead.

# PART TWO

# EAT

# CHAPTER 3:

# THE SIGNIFICANCE OF FOOD

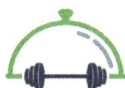

## A journey of discovery: Introducing my son to the world of food

As a parent, witnessing the milestones in my child's life has been a memorable journey filled with joy, wonder and sometimes, a touch of apprehension. One such milestone that stands out vividly in my memory is the moment my son experienced his first taste of solid food.

The fourth month of his life was a major milestone. Up until then, milk had been his sole source of nourishment, but it was evident that his growing body was craving more nutrition-dense food. He seemed constantly hungry, devouring his milk with lightning speed only to hunger again shortly after. The time had come to introduce him to the world of flavours beyond milk.

*With a spoonful of fruit puree, I approached him cautiously, unsure of his reaction. His initial response was a mixture of curiosity and uncertainty. His tiny fists clenched, his body tensed and his eyes widened in surprise as the foreign sensation hit his taste buds. I could almost sense his internal dialogue: "What is this?" His lips puckered, his tongue darted in and out and for a moment, I feared he might choke. But then, a spark of intrigue lit up his eyes and he leaned in, eager to explore this newfound alien taste.*

In the weeks that followed, we were both thrilled to explore various types of food together. From oranges to strawberries, bread to pasta, carrots to broccoli, there was no food he wouldn't try. And much to my delight, he devoured each one completely.

It was a heartwarming experience to witness his growing appreciation for the diverse flavours and textures that the world of food has to offer. Each mealtime was a cherished moment of discovery that bonded us as we experimented with new tastes and sensations.

Through it all, one thing became abundantly clear – my son and I shared not only a deep connection but also a mutual love for the sensory delight that good food has to offer.

Back when I was a teenager, I absolutely loved eating all kinds of food, until a few things happened that made me see food in a different light. I can still picture those high school hallways as if it were yesterday. Some of my classmates seemed to glide through them effortlessly, as though they belonged on a fashion runway. They had perfect bodies, like the models you see in magazines. Among them was my best friend who stood six feet tall with flawless skin and a slender figure. A real runway model, she had already confidently walked down catwalks. And then there was me.

Me? I was different. I was short and chubby, and I felt completely out of place next to all those seemingly perfect people. It made me start thinking differently about myself and the relationship I had with food.

As I navigated the insecurities of adolescence, the harsh whispers and snide remarks of girls seated at the back of the classroom, such as *"Are you sure you can fit through that door?"* became a constant voice in my head. Their words cut deep, leaving behind wounds that festered with self-doubt. I began to internalise their judgments, scrutinising every curve and imperfection I saw reflected in the mirror.

Fuelled by a desire to conform to their standards of beauty, I started my own research towards what I believed was the path to self-acceptance: weight loss. Armed with newfound knowledge gleaned from countless hours of research, I immersed myself in the world of calorie counting, carefully tracking every mouthful that passed my lips.

Each day was a relentless cycle of numbers: calories in, calories out. I obsessed over food labels, constantly recalculating my daily intake. Guilt accompanied every indulgence, reminding me of my never-ending quest for an elusive perfection. Though small progress eventually came, it wasn't as swift as I had hoped.

# CHAPTER 4:

# UNVEILING THE POWER OF CALORIES

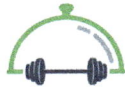

Food is the fuel that ignites the engine of our bodies. Just as cars require fuel to run and houses need electricity and gas to power appliances, our bodies rely on food for energy. At the heart of this energy exchange lies a fundamental concept: calories.

Calories represent the units of energy contained in the foods we eat. Each mouthful we consume translates into the energy needed to fuel our daily activities, from the mundane to the extraordinary. Every movement we make, whether it's blinking our eyes, walking, running, or simply standing tall, relies on the energy stored in our food.

Discovering the truth about calories was a revelation that reshaped my perspective on food and helped me gain control over my insecurities and tackle my body weight head-on. Armed with this knowledge, I understood the basics of calories. Within just a few weeks of diligently tracking my intake, I found myself effortlessly attuned to the caloric content of my meals. Little did I know that this newfound awareness would forever alter the trajectory of my life, leaving an indelible mark on my journey towards health and wellness.

Every morsel of food and sip of drink, with the exception of water, contributes to our daily caloric intake. Even seemingly innocuous choices, like a glass of lemon water, contain calories that contribute to our overall energy balance. The sum total of the calories we consume in a day determines the energy available to sustain us through our daily endeavours.

Yet, understanding our individual caloric needs can be difficult. Much like a growing infant whose appetite expands with each milestone reached, our caloric requirements fluctuate in response to factors such as age, gender, weight and physical activity level.

Consider the journey of my son during his infancy. In his earliest days, his sole source of sustenance was breastmilk, providing him with the energy needed for growth and development. As he grew, his caloric needs surged to accommodate for his growing body and the increased energy required for milestones like sitting up, standing and eventually crawling around the house like a vigilant security guard. Breastmilk alone could no longer suffice, prompting the introduction of purees, followed by baby cereal, to satiate his growing hunger. As he continued to grow and his metabolism raced to keep pace with his boundless energy, protein-rich foods like rice pudding, chicken, eggs and hearty pasta became staples of his diet. With each passing week and month, his portion sizes expanded to fuel his insatiable appetite for exploration and discovery.

For adults, tools such as an energy needs calculator provided by reputable sources like The Eat for Health[2] website offers invaluable guidance in determining our daily energy requirements. By inputting variables such as age, gender, weight and activity level, we gain insight into the optimal caloric intake needed to support our individual lifestyles.

# Decoding calories

To measure my caloric intake, I armed myself with a charming diary. With each meal and snack carefully recorded, my food diary became my newfound dedication to understanding the intricacies of calories.

An example of a day in my diary;

| Breakfast was two eggs | XX calories |
|---|---|
| A slice of toast | X calories |
| A cup of milk coffee | X calories |
| Lunch | XXX calories |
| Dinner | XXX calories |
| Desserts | XXX calories |
| **Total calorie consumption** | **XXXXXX** |

Turning to the internet for guidance, I discovered the caloric content of every item I consumed, diligently noting down the energy value "X" for every food I consumed in a day. As the day drew to a close, I assigned a numerical score to each food, transforming my meals into a mathematical equation. The sum total '"XXXXX", a final figure at the end of the day provided me with insight into the total number of calories I consumed that day. This means that any excess calories I consumed were stored as fat.

As I dived deeper into this newfound practice, I eventually excelled at the precision with which I could decipher the rough caloric content of my meals. What once seemed like a daunting task soon became second nature. In a matter of days, I could effortlessly tally my daily intake in less than two minutes with consistency and dedication. In a matter of months, I did not even require a diary as I subconsciously kept track of the quantity intake in my mind.

Just like a mathematician, I knew the maths would work if I paid attention to my calories like an equation.

| Daily consumption  <  Daily requirement  = Calorie Deficit (Weight Loss) |
| --- |
| Daily consumption  >  Daily requirement  = Calorie Surplus (Weight Gain) |
| Daily consumption  =  Daily calorie requirement (Maintain Weight) |

Our bodies store excess calories as fat when the energy is not utilised, acting like a vault to ensure reserves are available for future needs. When we increase our physical activity or maintain a calorie deficit, these stored fats are converted back into energy, facilitating fat loss. However, fat loss is often accompanied by muscle loss, which can be mitigated by incorporating strength training into our routines during the fat loss process.

For those aiming to increase their body mass, weight training while maintaining a calorie surplus with high-quality food will lead to great results to gain weight. Therefore, calorie tracking is a crucial tool for both weight loss and weight gain, allowing us to effectively manage our energy balance and achieve our desired body composition goals.

In my weight loss journey during adolescence, I diligently tracked my consumption, all the while harbouring a desire to trim my excess weight. With each entry, I scrutinised my choices, seeking opportunities to make subtle yet impactful adjustments. A slice of toast eliminated, a switch from full-fat with low-fat milk, a trade-off from deep-fried indulgences to lighter fare — each modification chipped away at my daily caloric intake.

Initially, the results of my efforts remained elusive. Despite my best intentions, the numbers on the scale refused to budge. Yet, I persevered, trusting in the power of small changes to yield significant outcomes. Much like Warren Buffett's strategy of making small but consistent efforts for long-term investing emphasises the importance of patience and persistence for a compounding effect. I applied the same principles to my journey toward health and wellness. Each adjustment to my diet, no matter how modest, contributed to the cumulative effect of progress over time.

And then, like a beacon of hope in the night sky, progress emerged after several months. In the quiet moments of reflection, I witnessed the subtle transformations taking place within my body. The once-elusive goal of weight loss began to materialise before my eyes due to my consistency and determination. It must be noted that weight changes cannot be too drastic. If you are aiming to lose weight, aim to lose no more than half a kilogram per week. The slower we make the changes, the longer they last without compromising our health.

As days turned into several weeks, my relationship with food underwent a profound shift. No longer bound by the confines of my diary, I had developed an intuitive understanding of my dietary needs. The act of journaling evolved into a subconscious skill, allowing me to navigate the complexities of caloric intake with ease. With newfound confidence, I embraced the concept of a weekly indulgence — a cheat day, if you will — where I allowed myself to indulge in any food without restraint. Yet, even amidst the decadence, I remained mindful of the delicate balance between indulgence and restraint, ensuring that my weekly excesses were offset by disciplined moderation on other days. Without realising I had shifted my daily tracking to weekly tracking in my mind without the need to write in a journal.

In this intricate dance of calories and cravings, I discovered the true essence of balance. By harnessing the power of mathematics to unravel the puzzle of my diet, I unlocked a pathway to lasting health and wellness. Fast forward 27 years from then to now and I am still reaping the benefits of the calorie tracking skills I honed all those years ago in my teenage days. Through the ups and downs of life's journey, from the joys of pregnancy to the challenges of postpartum recovery, I have relied on these foundational principles to navigate the ever-changing landscape of my health and weight. With each passing year, I have adapted and refined my approach, drawing upon the lessons learned to maintain my fitness and achieve my ideal weight. As I reflect on the decades that have shaped me, I am grateful for the simple yet profound wisdom that continues to guide me toward a lifetime of maintaining my ideal weight.

There is indeed great power in understanding the caloric needs of our bodies. However, the question remains: is it enough to rely solely on calories to sustain us? The answer lies in the broader concept of nutrition. While calories provide the energy necessary to fuel our daily activities, nutrition encompasses much more than mere energy provision.

Nutrition delves into the quality of the calories we consume, exploring the vital role that nutrients play in supporting our overall health and well-being.

# CHAPTER 5:

# NUTRITION: EAT FOR HEALTH

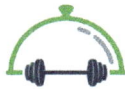

In the bustling rhythm of modern life, where convenience often takes precedence over nutritional value, it's easy to overlook the importance of what we fuel our bodies with. Yet, beneath the surface of our daily routines, it's easy to overlook that our bodies depend on a balanced and varied diet to thrive.

Imagine your body as a finely tuned machine, requiring a specific blend of fuels to operate at its best. While calories serve as the currency of energy, nutrition provides the blueprint for optimal health and vitality. Our bodies are intricate and dynamic, demanding more than just basic sustenance. They crave nourishment in the form of vitamins, minerals, proteins, carbohydrates and fats — a symphony of nutrients working in harmony to sustain life itself.

But why does nutrition matter? Beyond satisfying hunger pangs and filling our bellies, the foods we choose to consume play a pivotal role in shaping our health trajectory. A balanced and wholesome diet not only fuels our physical endeavours but may also serve as a potent shield against disease and chronic ailments. A good and balanced diet forms the bedrock of disease prevention and vitality. By incorporating a diverse array of nutrient-rich foods into our meals, we provide our bodies with the essential tools they need to thrive.

Conversely, poor dietary choices high in saturated fats, refined sugars and processed foods can contribute to inflammation, weight gain and an increased susceptibility to illness.

With my conscious calorie balancing act, I believed I had finally gained mastery over the relationship between food and my body. Through careful monitoring and mindful consumption, I had managed to achieve some fat loss and the once harsh comments from colleagues had gradually faded into silence. It appears I had cracked the code to optimal nutrition, but little did I know, this was only half the picture.

As I continued my journey towards better health, I found solace in activities that kept me moving, from swimming laps in the early morning to tending to household chores with vigour. These newfound habits, coupled with my vigilant calorie counting, propelled me toward my goals, inch by inch, pound by pound.

It was almost a decade later, amidst the hustle and bustle of office life, that I stumbled upon a revelation that would forever alter my perspective on nutrition. Enticed by the promise of a free gym membership offered by my workplace, I ventured into the world of strength training — an endeavour that would not only transform my physique but also ignite a newfound curiosity about the quality of the fuel I was providing my body.

As I toiled away amidst the clanking of weights and the dances of exercise classes, I found myself drawn to the deeper intricacies of food and its impact on our bodies. No longer content with merely counting calories, I began to dig deeper into food quality, seeking to unravel the mysteries of macronutrients and micronutrients. It was a revelation that shook me to my core, challenging my preconceived notions about the role of food in our lives.

# Eat for health Australian guide

In the array of food resources, there lies a source of nutritional wisdom, a guiding light in healthy eating: Eat for Health. Eat for Health isn't just any website; it's an initiative by the Australian Government, demonstrating a commitment to the health and well-being of its citizens and anyone seeking guidance on food nutrition. With its treasure trove of information on food and nutrition, it stands as a powerful source of knowledge in shaping healthier lifestyles.

The website provides guidelines that empower individuals to learn about food and nutrition. From calorie calculators that demystify the often-perplexing world of energy intake to comprehensive dietary guidelines that serve as a roadmap to balanced nutrition, Eat for Health promotes guidelines for healthier eating habits.

One of the most helpful guides is the concept of food groups. By categorising foods into five distinct groups, each representing a vital component of a balanced diet, Eat for Health provides a framework for making informed choices about what we put on our plates.

**Group 1 - Grain (cereal) foods**: This group forms the foundation of a healthy diet, with an emphasis on whole grains (cereal) that provide essential nutrients, fibre and a good source of complex carbohydrates.

**Group 2 - Vegetables and legumes/beans:** Bursting with vitamins, minerals and antioxidants.

**Group 3 - Lean meats and poultry, fish, eggs, tofu, nuts, seeds and legumes/beans:** Protein-rich foods are the building blocks of a strong and healthy body, and this group provides them in abundance.

**Group 4 - Milk, yoghurt, cheese and/or alternatives**, mostly reduced fat, which are rich in calcium and protein.

**Group 5 - Fruits:** Nature's sweetest bounty, fruits are a treasure trove of vitamins, minerals and fibre.

The Australian Guide to Healthy Eating is a one-page printable guide that recommends enjoying a wide variety of nutritious foods from the above five food groups daily, to stay hydrated with plenty of water and to limit alcohol and highly processed foods for healthy eating[3].

Limiting processed foods is a smart approach to a sustainable and healthy diet. While it is possible to adhere to a highly restrictive healthy eating plan for a short period, this is often not sustainable in the long term. Eating habits are lifelong and the key to maintaining them is to have a balance. By limiting processed foods to once a week or even once a month, you create a realistic and achievable diet that you are more likely to stick to.

The less food is handled and processed, the healthier it tends to be. That is why home-cooked meals are generally a better choice than fast food. For instance, a homemade meal involves minimal processing compared to a fast-food burger, which goes through numerous stages of preparation, reducing its nutritional value. Therefore, adopting a balanced approach that emphasises whole, minimally processed foods can lead to better health and more sustainable eating habits.

# CHAPTER 6:

# UNDERSTANDING MACRO AND MICRO NUTRITION

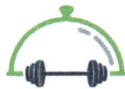

## Macronutrition

Macronutrition is the building blocks of life that take centre stage, fuelling our bodies with the energy needed to sustain life itself.

Macronutrition refers to nutrition at a higher level, focusing on the food required in larger quantities, hence the term "macro". It is an exploration of the fundamental components of our diet that contribute to our daily energy intake. Yet, not all sources of energy are created equal. While alcohol and junk food may indeed provide us with a surge of calories, they fall short in fulfilling the nutritional needs required to sustain life.

Macronutrition has three main components — proteins, fats and carbohydrates — that form the backbone of our dietary landscape. Each macronutrient plays a unique role in fuelling our bodies, providing the energy needed to power our daily endeavours and maintain optimal health.

# The power of proteins in macronutrition

Proteins, often hailed as the "king of macronutrients," serve as the foundation upon which our bodies are constructed. From the muscles that propel us forward to the enzymes that catalyse vital biochemical reactions, proteins play a pivotal role in nearly every aspect of our physiology. Found abundantly in sources such as meat, fish, poultry, eggs and dairy products, these essential nutrients provide the amino acids needed to support muscle repair, immune function and hormone regulation.

For gym-goers and bodybuilders alike, proteins hold a special place as they promise bigger, stronger muscles and enhanced athletic performance. Indeed, the role of proteins in supporting muscle repair and growth cannot be overstated, making them a favourite among fitness enthusiasts seeking to optimise their physical prowess.

The recommended protein intake is 1 gram per kilogram of the bodyweight. So, if you weigh 70 kg you should eat around 70 grams of protein per day[4]. This avoids over consumption of protein and too much red meat consumption can increase the risk of heart disease. Hence, it's important to obtain protein from a variety of sources. Protein takes longer to digest than other nutrients, which helps you feel fuller for longer periods and aids in managing your appetite.

# Embracing the vitality of healthy fats

In the midst of the chaos during my IVF treatments, I stumbled upon an old tale that promised the birth of intelligent babies that walnuts produced. With each passing day of my pregnancy, I clung to this tale with utter devotion, determined to bestow upon my child the gift of intelligence and wisdom.

And so, amidst the morning sickness of my pregnancy, I faithfully consumed walnuts with unwavering dedication. Even in the darkest depths of extreme sickness, when my stomach rebelled against all forms of sustenance, I persisted by shoving handfuls of walnuts into my mouth. As my pregnancy progressed, I made a curious observation: the stark contrast between pre-packaged walnuts, with their pungent odour and stale taste and freshly cracked walnuts, imbued with the earthy fragrance of vitality and freshness.

When my son was finally born, the size of his head fell towards the larger end of the spectrum. The tiny beanies I packed in my hospital bag were all too small to fit his head. A year later, as daycare teachers noticed his cleverness for his age, I couldn't help but wonder if it was the miracle of the walnuts that had contributed to his intelligence.

Though I may never know for certain, one thing remains clear: Fats, the healthy ones, help our bodies absorb nutrients. Found in a variety of forms, from heart-healthy unsaturated fats found in nuts, seeds and avocados to the essential fatty acids abundant in fatty fish, these dietary fats provide the energy needed to fuel our daily endeavours while supporting cognitive function and nutrient absorption. Healthy oils for cooking, for example, olive, canola, sunflower, peanut and soybean oil. These foods can help lower your cholesterol[5].

## Carbohydrates: Navigating a complex relationship

And then there are carbohydrates, the primary source of energy for our bodies and make up a significant portion of our macronutrition. In my opinion, it is also the double-edged sword of the dietary world, capable of both energising and becoming the enemy for fat loss.

In the intricate dance of nutrition, I found myself in a love-hate relationship with carbohydrates also called carbs. As the descendants of farmers on my mother's side, carbs loomed large in my upbringing, their presence pervasive in our family's diet. From steaming bowls of rice to hearty servings of potatoes and flatbread, carbs formed the backbone of every meal, providing the energy needed to fuel our daily endeavours. Yet, as I watched my mother and her siblings grapple with a myriad of health issues, belly fat, from diabetes to heart disease, all stemming from over consumption of carbs and a sedentary lifestyle, I couldn't help but question the role carbs played in our family's well-being.

It was a realisation born of necessity that there existed a direct relationship between carbs and physical energy expenditure. During the arduous days spent toiling on the farm, my ancestors relied heavily on carbs to sustain them through long hours of physical labour, their bodies demanding a constant and quick influx of energy to fuel their physical exertion.

And yet, as I navigated my own journey towards health and vitality, I discovered that the relationship between carbs and energy was far more nuanced than I had ever imagined. Consuming carbs a day or a few hours before an intense training session, I found myself endowed with newfound strength and stamina, able to push harder and reach new heights of physical performance at the gym. It was as if carbs acted as a potent fuel, igniting my muscles with the energy needed to achieve peak performance. Amidst the turmoil of conflicting emotions, I began to uncover a glimmer of understanding — a realisation that carbs are not inherently good or bad. Instead, their impact on our bodies largely depends on context and timing. In fact, I experienced the most significant gains in muscle size and strength when I increased my carbs along with my protein intake.

I discovered the intricate dance between carbs and energy metabolism. Carbs, I learned, serve as the primary source of fuel for our bodies, providing the glucose needed to power our muscles and sustain our physical endeavours. For a family of farmers, whose livelihoods depended on long hours of strenuous labour in the fields, it made sense that carbs would feature prominently in our diet, providing the energy needed to work the land and reap its bounty. The amount of carbs required is directly related to the intensity of the physical activity. The key is to find the subtle balance and load up with most of the intake around the training sessions. Since carbs are easily processed, they provide an instant energy to power through training sessions. On the other hand, they can also easily convert to fats if not expended as energy.

Many fitness enthusiasts promote low-carb diets. Yet, as I forged a path towards a balanced approach to nutrition, I learned to embrace carbs not as the enemy, but as a vital component of a healthy diet that helps me with my strength and stamina. From my favourite oats, rice and legumes to fruits and vegetables, I discovered a diverse array of wholemeal carbohydrate-rich foods that provided sustained energy and nourishment without the accompanying spikes in blood sugar. I also learned to consume more carbs before my workouts and afterward to give me an extra boost of energy.

In the end, it is not the carbs themselves that determine your fate but rather, the mindful choices we make in how, when and what type we consume and utilise this essential nutrient. Stick to quality carbs such as wholemeal grains, rice, oats, pasta and potatoes. Consume the bulk of them before your training sessions, ideally a day or few hours before, to get more out of your training sessions. Carbs are also a brain food so an extreme low-carbs diet can make you fatigued and weak. Hence, try not to cut too much carbs from your diet.

From the complex carbs found in whole grains, fruits and vegetables to the simple sugars found in honey and maple syrup, carbs provide the fuel needed to power our daily activities and metabolic processes. Yet, amidst the abundance of sources of carbs that adorn our plates, it is crucial to prioritise quality over quantity, opt for nutrient-dense sources that provide sustained energy without the accompanying spikes in blood sugar.

# Micronutrition

Contrary to macronutrients, micronutrients such as vitamins and minerals operate behind the scenes, performing an array of essential functions. Our bodies require only a small number of micronutrients, which is why they are labelled as "micro".

In the grand narrative of sustenance, these tiny warriors play a crucial role, despite their modest presence in our diets. While their counterparts, the macronutrients, dominate the stage with their bulk and energy, it is the micronutrients that quietly orchestrate the intricate dance of cellular processes within our bodies. They are the unsung facilitators, enabling the body to produce enzymes, hormones and other vital substances necessary for the symphony of life. Without their tuned choreography, our growth and development would falter, and the harmonious balance of our internal ecosystem would be disrupted.

But despite their microscopic stature, the impact of micronutrients on our well-being is monumental. A deficiency in any of these nutrients can compromise health, leading to a cascade of debilitating consequences. From weakened immune systems to impaired cognitive function, the repercussions of micronutrient deficiencies can be severe and, in some cases, life-threatening[6].

There are several essential micronutrients, such as Vitamins A, B, C, D, E and K, along with various minerals like calcium, iron, magnesium and zinc[7]. These micronutrients play diverse roles in various bodily processes, from supporting immune function to aiding in metabolism and growth.

In a world inundated with quick-fix diets and fleeting food trends, it is easy to lose sight of the importance of a well-balanced diet. Yet, it is through the harmonious interplay of a diverse array of foods that we obtain the full spectrum of micronutrients our bodies crave. Fruits, vegetables, legumes, whole grains, lean proteins and healthy fats — all are essential players in this nutritional orchestra, each contributing its unique repertoire of micronutrients to the symphony of health.

For me, the allure of fad diets has always been overshadowed by the wisdom of balance and moderation. These trendy regimens, with their promises of rapid transformation, often come at a cost, slashing away entire food groups and inadvertently depriving us of vital micronutrients. There are no shortcuts on the path to vitality; only the steadfast commitment to nourish the body with the wholesome abundance it deserves.

## Antioxidants and fibre

Eating food comes naturally to me, but ensuring I consume enough servings of fruits and vegetables is always the real challenge. Our bodies age every passing day, much like how oxygen corrodes iron. While oxygen sustains our lives, it also generates free radicals that harm cells, proteins and DNA[8]. Antioxidants play a crucial role in neutralising these free radicals, safeguarding our cellular integrity. Therefore, it is evident that incorporating plenty of fruits and vegetables into our daily diet is essential for ageing gracefully.

One part of our diet that is often overlooked is the role of dietary fibre, found in vegetables, fruits, bran and whole grains. It is like the unsung hero of our meals. Its presence, more than just a dietary component, shapes the delicate balance of our internal ecosystem.

Dietary fibre means that fraction of the edible parts of plants or their extracts, or synthetic analogues, that are indigestible that our bodies can't break down completely. Instead, it travels through our system, sweeping away waste and keeping things moving along[9].

Now, why is this important? Well, a well-functioning gut means better digestion and better absorption of nutrients from the food we eat. Plus, fibre acts like a superhero for our gut bacteria. It's their favourite food! When they munch on fibre, they produce helpful compounds that benefit our overall physical and mental health[10]. Consuming a wide variety of fruits and vegetables can enhance this microbial ecosystem, as different types of fibre nourish various beneficial bacteria. By expanding your diet to include a rich assortment of fresh fruits and vegetables, you can promote a healthier and more robust gut microbiome, which in turn, supports the overall digestive health and well-being.

From the age of six months, I made a concerted effort to introduce my son to a diverse array of fresh fruits and vegetables. Whether it was offering cucumber sticks to soothe his gums or tantalising his taste buds with plump strawberries, juicy watermelon, oranges, sticks of carrots and bushy broccoli, his tiny fingers eagerly explored each new flavour. It was a delightful journey for both of us as I eagerly anticipated each day introducing him to new foods.

On days when my energy ran low, I employed my trusted trick of sneaking finely chopped baby spinach into his omelettes or blending it into juices to enrich his pasta sauce. It's safe to say that he now relishes a wide variety of fruits and many vegetables, with vegetables usually being the first to be emptied from his plate. This proves the significance of early exposure to nutritious foods.

# CHAPTER 7:

# THE GIFT OF TASTE

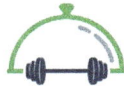

My journey into the world of food did not begin with grand ambitions or gourmet aspirations. It was a path forged through the trials of long university hours and the demands of professional life. Throughout my twenties, my days were consumed by studies and work, leaving little room to savour the delights of the palate. For years, meals were merely sustenance, serving to an end in the pursuit of knowledge and career aspirations. It wasn't until fate intervened in the form of a chance encounter with my now ex-husband that my perception of food underwent a profound transformation.

In the busy corridors of our workplace, amidst the hum of fluorescent lights and the noises of keyboards, our paths converged. He loved to cook and his passion for food inspired me. Hailing from England, his family's love affair with cooking went beyond basic nourishment, elevating food into an art and a source of family joy, connection and endless discovery.

Unlike most men I had encountered, his enthusiasm for creating and savouring delectable dishes stood out. Our early years together were a whirlwind of food exploration, as we embraced a prolonged honeymoon phase that spanned across continents and cultures.

From the prestigious dining rooms of London's Alain Ducasse At The Dorchester, a three Michelin stars illuminated our palates with masterpieces, to the rustic charm of Tuscany's secluded villages in a vineyard, where humble eggplant ravioli and handcrafted pasta captured the essence of Italian cuisine – each destination offered a unique culinary adventure.

Our quest for culinary enlightenment didn't stop there. We found ourselves wandering the bustling streets of Thailand, indulging in freshly hand-picked fish cooked to perfection by street vendors whose skilful hands transformed humble ingredients into delicious delights. In Lyon, France, known as the city of a thousand flavours, we dove into a cheese paradise, exploring through a diverse range of options that excited and expanded our taste buds.

For us, travel was not just about sightseeing; it was about tasting the world through its flavours - one dish at a time. Each meal became an opportunity to connect with a culture, uncovering the stories and traditions woven into the fabric of its cuisine. As we travelled the globe, I discovered a deep appreciation for exploring the diverse flavours of delicious cuisines.

Over the course of a decade spent exploring various foods with him, I learned a valuable lesson - that food is more than just fuel; it's a source of joy, connection and nourishment that sparks mindfulness tasting in every bite. I discovered the simplicity of flavourful dishes crafted from just a few ingredients. In a world inundated with excess, I found pure joy in the mindful consumption of delicious food, trusting that each bite nourished not only the body but the spirit as well.

Inspired by simplicity and flavour, I adopted Jamie Oliver's mantra of using just five ingredients to create wholesome and delicious meals in a fraction of the time. It was a revelation, a reminder that good food need not be complicated. With a few quality ingredients and a dash of creativity, anyone can become a great cook and create quick meals to fit our busy lives.

When the era of Covid-19 arrived, it brought with it a wave of unprecedented challenges, reshaping the fabric of our lives in ways we never imagined. As the relentless march of the pandemic reached its peak, I found myself among the countless individuals grappling with the harsh realities of Covid-19. The first week of my infection was a harrowing ordeal, characterised by fever, fatigue and a relentless cough that seemed to sap the very essence of my being. Yet, little did I know that the true test awaited me in the weeks that followed.

As the virus swept through our lives, leaving a trail of illness and uncertainty in its wake, I found myself grappling with its relentless grip. It was not until the insidious onset of anosmia and ageusia — the loss of smell and taste — that the true gravity of my situation dawned upon me. Six weeks of deprivation, six weeks of anguish and six weeks of utter despair as I struggled with the silent torment of losing two of my most cherished senses: smell and taste.

Gone were the fragrant wafts of jasmine flowers that once danced on the breeze, their intoxicating aroma a balm for the soul. In their absence, the world seemed dull and lifeless, a world which once illuminated my senses.

But perhaps the cruellest blow of all was the loss of taste, that sacred communion between the palate and the plate that had once brought me so much joy. Even the simplest of dishes, like the humble omelette, laid tasteless and uninspiring, a mere semblance of its former self. In those days, the world around me seemed muted, colourless, drained of vitality. I clung to that flicker of hope, navigating the shadows with steadfast determination, trusting that one day, the colours would return, the flavours would awaken, and life would once again be infused with the vibrancy it so richly deserves. Those six weeks felt like an eternity, and I vowed never to take my taste buds for granted again.

# Types of taste

Outlined by the Australian Academy of Science, the basic tastes, often referred to as primary tastes, encompass sweet, sour, salty, bitter and umami (savoury or meat)[11]. These tastes play a crucial role in our taste buds, aiding us in perceiving and relishing a diverse array of foods. Each taste serves a distinct purpose in our diet, enhancing our overall eating experience and contributing to our sense of satisfaction and nourishment.

**Sweetness** is associated with sugars and carbohydrates. It provides energy and helps us identify the sources of carbohydrates in our diet, such as fruits, grains and some vegetables.

**Sourness** comes from acids in foods and can indicate the presence of vitamins (like vitamin C) and other beneficial compounds. Sour tastes can stimulate salivation and aid digestion.

**Saltiness** is important for maintaining the balance of electrolyte in the body. It enhances the flavour of foods and helps us identify sources of essential minerals like sodium.

**Bitterness** can alert us to the presence of potentially harmful substances, such as toxins or spoiled foods. It can also add complexity and balance to flavours when present in moderation.

**Umami** is often described as savoury or meaty and is associated with the presence of glutamate, an amino acid. Umami enhances the overall flavour of foods and can make them more satisfying and enjoyable to eat.

By discerning and appreciating these basic tastes, we can make informed dietary decisions, embrace a diverse and balanced diet and derive pleasure and fulfilment from our meals. By incorporating a variety of these tastes, we not only heighten our overall eating experience but also contribute to our sense of satisfaction and nourishment, making every meal both enjoyable and fulfilling.

After fully recovering from COVID-19, I found myself sitting in quiet contemplation, savouring the return of my senses. My heart swelled with gratitude for the simple pleasures that life offered. With each breath, I embraced a profound appreciation for the world around me. Closing my eyes, I whispered a silent promise – to cherish every taste, every moment, as if it were my last. In the midst of this symphony of sensation, I uncovered the true essence of life, a delicate balance of beauty and fragility that reminded me of the preciousness of each moment we are given.

# PART THREE

# TRAIN

# CHAPTER 8:

# THE PATH TO FITNESS

As I gazed at my reflection in the mirror, adorned in my princess-like ivory-white wedding dress with flawless makeup and hair, I couldn't help but be delighted at the surreal moment unfolding before me. How could I, an ordinary woman, be blessed with such an extraordinary fortune?

The wedding aisle stretched before me, presented a rustic charm and delicate details that painted a picture of my dream come true. It was an outdoor rustic wedding surrounded by white baby's breath, where paper butterflies fluttered out of the books at each table. The burlap roses almost seemed to carry the scent of real roses and numerous jars were neatly wrapped with burlap ribbons featuring cute buttons of all sizes with candles tucked between the whitest sand. Each detail, which I had gently handcrafted over the course of six months, spoke volumes of the love and dedication

I poured into preparing for the most significant day of my life to start a lifetime together with the man I loved.

And yet, amidst the joy and anticipation, there lingered a sense of disbelief — was this truly my reality? Had I truly found my happily ever after? With my demanding and seemingly endless education complete, alongside a stable career and my devoted long-term partner at my side, I stood on the brink of a new chapter, filled with love, hope and the promise of starting a new family together for a perfect loving family. But little did I know that the path I was about to tread would lead me into the eye of a storm, forever altering the course of my life.

Just weeks after pledging our vows before friends and family, my world was shattered by the revelation that my newlywed husband no longer loved me and that the wedding was his mistake. His confession was a dagger to my heart, a betrayal of the trust we had solemnly pledged before our loved ones. In any other circumstance, anger or screams might have been the natural response, but I was rendered speechless by the sudden, unexpected trauma. The euphoria of starting a new chapter in life crashed down right before me in mere seconds, leaving me reeling in disbelief. All I could do was sit there like a frozen statue, paralyzed by the weight of this heartbreaking revelation. Just as I thought my life was having a fairytale beginning, life has a funny way of reminding us we are least in control.

The aftermath of his abrupt abandonment plunged me into the darkest period of my life. I found myself grappling with a loss unlike any other, a loss that I wasn't prepared for in any shape or form. I felt like a widow mourning the loss of her spouse, whose husband still walked among the living. The emptiness consumed me, suffocating me with its relentless grip. I sat like a lifeless piece of furniture in an empty room while life passed by. The only reminder of my own existence was that I was breathing. It was a surreal and excruciating truth that I struggled to comprehend for months. Appetite became a distant memory and eating turned into a daunting task. Tears flowed endlessly, causing a constant ache in my stomach. He had lifted me to great heights, promising a bright future together, only to ruthlessly thrust me into the chilling depths below, where loneliness engulfed me like a suffocating cloak.

Lost in the depths, my limbs felt tied, leaving me unable to climb up to rescue myself or find another path to take to escape the depths of that bottomless pit. Words of consolation from those who deeply cared about me could be seen leaving their mouths, yet somehow, they skipped my processing ability, their words only to be converted to a distant mumble seeping through a long, dark tunnel. The very sound of weddings that once got me excited, now even their mention or a sight of pregnant women who passed by was excruciatingly painful to watch as they served as a reminder of the family, I had dreamed of but may never have. Yet, amidst the despair, I knew deep down that I had to find a way forward to survive.

Forced to confront my mental health head-on, I pushed myself to explore new avenues in search of solace and healing. I immersed myself in trying things that sparked even the slightest hint of joy. From experimenting with makeup techniques to testing the world of language with Spanish lessons, I embraced every opportunity for growth and renewal. Reconnecting with my passion for fitness, I pushed myself to new limits, using physical exertion as a means of overcoming the deep emotional wounds.

In the midst of heartbreak and despair, I emerged as a stronger, more resilient version of myself. Though the scars of betrayal may never fully heal, I refused to let them define me. Instead, I chose to embrace the pain as a catalyst for transformation, forging a path toward a brighter, more hopeful future.

## Selecting the ideal fitness regimen

Finding the ideal fitness regimen is similar to setting out on a quest for the perfect meal. Just as you can't truly know the flavours you will savour until you take that first bite, discovering the right type of fitness requires exploration, experimentation and a willingness to try new things. However, before taking that first step, it is paramount to seek guidance from a health or exercise professional, especially if you are inactive, pregnant, your fitness level is low, or have never exercised before.

Reflecting on the early days of nurturing my newborn son, while eating and sleeping came naturally to him, his tiny frame often battled the discomfort of gas. In the newborn stage, it was recommended that I guide him through exercises like tummy time and the gentle cycling of his legs, actions designed not just to aid digestion but to help him build his strength. My conscious intervention was required for his physical development, as he was mostly inactive in the newborn stage. But as he grew into toddlerhood, the need for such conscious intervention was no longer required. Running, jumping, climbing and sometimes even punching were his normal activities, which are the natural human movements ingrained in us all from birth.

And yet, for many adults, we may find that eating and sleeping come as naturally as drawing breath, yet the conscious decision to engage in physical activity remains a deliberate choice. In a world where convenience often trumps conscious choice and due to our modern sedentary lifestyle, the pursuit of physical fitness becomes a deliberate act, a commitment to reclaiming the vigour that lies dormant within us. Our bodies only function efficiently by staying active.

The key to unlocking the ideal fitness regimen lies in finding an activity that resonates with you on a deep level — one that ignites your passion and leaves you feeling both invigorated and refreshed. It's about finding something that allows you to disconnect from the stresses of the world while simultaneously rejuvenating your spirit, leaving you ready to tackle whatever life throws your way. When it comes to selecting the perfect fitness regimen, there are a few important factors to consider. First and foremost, it's crucial to find an activity that aligns with your lifestyle and preferences. Whether you prefer the tranquillity of yoga or the adrenaline rush of high-intensity interval training, the key is to choose something that feels like a natural extension of who you are.

Additionally, it's essential to consider the intensity level of your chosen activity. While some may thrive on the challenge of pushing their physical limits, others may prefer a more moderate approach. There's no right or wrong answer — what matters most is finding a level of intensity that feels sustainable and enjoyable for you. Your fitness journey isn't about reaching a specific destination but rather embracing an evolving identity — one where your chosen activities become an integral part of who you are to form your identity. Furthermore, don't be afraid to explore a variety of different fitness options. Just as you wouldn't limit yourself to eating the same meal every day, there's no need to confine yourself to just one type of exercise. Whether it's yoga on Monday, strength training on Wednesday, or a dance class on Friday, mixing things up can help keep your workouts interesting and engaging.

Personally, I've ventured down numerous paths in search of the perfect fitness regimen. From attempting gymnastics, which demanded a level of flexibility I no longer possessed, to aerobic classes that left me feeling queasy and even boxing, where my lack of coordination proved to be a stumbling block, I explored a wide range of options in pursuit of my fitness goals. However, it wasn't until I discovered the transformative power of strength, resistance or weight training that I truly found my stride. Not only did strength training provide me with a challenging yet attainable workout, but it also served as a catalyst for unlocking a new chapter in my journey toward healing and redemption.

In the chapters that follow, I will share with you my experiences, insights and discoveries of self-discovery and transformation through the world of strength training. What began as a simple endeavour to nourish my mind and spirit soon blossomed into a profound exploration of my body's capabilities. With each rep, each set and each milestone reached, I found myself awestruck by the incredible changes unfolding within me — changes that defied the limitations I once believed were limited to my genetics. Through sweat and determination, I witnessed my body sculpt and strengthen, resulting in the power of resilience and perseverance. Along the way, I'll share the insights and revelations that I learned from my journey, offering guidance and inspiration for those who want to follow their own path to strength training and emotional well-being.

# Benefits of strength training

One of the unique advantages for beginners who want to start strength training is that fat loss and muscle growth can go hand in hand in the first few years. Unlike advanced trainers, who must often prioritise fat loss or muscle gain, beginners enjoy the best of both worlds without making compromises. This phenomenon makes the early stages of strength training a golden opportunity not to be missed.

There are two types of training: cardiovascular, often referred to as cardio and strength, resistance, or weight training. I hear countless debates about whether one should concentrate on cardio to lose weight and avoid strength training, while others advocate solely focusing on weights and skipping cardio altogether. But the reality is that both have their rightful place in a well-rounded fitness program.

Cardio involves activities that raise your heart rate, keep it elevated for the duration of the workout and keep your heart muscles functioning well. Whether you're running, cycling, or swimming, cardio challenges your cardiovascular system, forcing your heart to work harder and become more efficient at pumping blood throughout your body. This leads to a stronger heart and improved cardiovascular health. Additionally, cardio burns calories while you're performing the activity, making it an effective tool for weight management.

However, it's important to note that the calorie burn during cardio is typically lower compared to a session of strength training.

Now, let's shift our focus to strength or resistance training, which involves weights or resistance to build strength in your muscles. Unlike cardio, which primarily burns calories during the activity itself, strength training offers a unique advantage: it continues to burn calories even after the session has ended. This after-burn effect means that your body continues to expend energy as it repairs and rebuilds muscle tissue in the hours and days following a strength training workout — even while you sleep! This makes strength training a powerful tool for not only building muscle but also for boosting metabolism and promoting fat loss over the long term.

But here's the catch: true magic happens when you combine the two. By incorporating both cardio and strength training into your fitness routine, you create a powerful synergy that maximises results. Cardio strengthens your heart and improves endurance, while strength training builds muscle mass and makes you strong.

Together, they form a potent combination that accelerates fat loss, improves overall fitness and enhances cardiovascular health. By integrating both modalities into your fitness routine, you unlock the full spectrum of benefits, ensuring a balanced approach to fitness that strengthens not only your body but also your heart and mind.

Some of the benefits of strength training are increased strength and muscular endurance, effective weight management, maintaining flexibility and balance, boosting energy levels and mood, increasing bone density and preventing falls and fractures[12]. Through my personal journey with strength training, I have unearthed a multitude of benefits. Notably, the profound impact on my self-confidence and mental well-being has been nothing short of transformative. The weight of depression and anxiety, once an anchor dragging me into the depths of despair, began to lift, replaced by a sense of calm and clarity that I had never felt.

Initially, the noticeable changes were internal: an improved mood, better sleep quality, management of depression and anxiety and an appetite for healthy food. As consistency became my thing, the physical transformations followed suit. Rounded shoulders, a hallmark of years spent hunched over a corporate desk, gave way to a proud posture. The grip of gravity on my chest that once caused saggy boobs was lifted and my waistline gradually toned. With each session, I defied not only gravity but also the limitations imposed by genetics, sculpting a body that is proportionate to my height. Though it took me roughly two years to see some significant results since I didn't know what I was doing in the first few years, this book has solely been to help and inspire those who want to start or have just started training. I realised that achieving your desired body weight isn't solely about food and nutrition, which are still half of its secrets; it's also about understanding through strength training you can effectively control your body's energy expenditure.

CHAPTER 9:

# THINGS TO CONSIDER BEFORE BEGINNING TRAINING

Before we begin the intricacies of strength training, it's imperative to address the prevalent misconception that training is solely the domain of a particular gender or age group. During my fitness journey, I have noticed a striking observation: roughly only 1 out of 10 people on the gym floor have been women who perform strength training, which shows that there exists a stark gender disparity. It's not uncommon to find a mere fraction of women amidst the sea of male counterparts, revealing a stigma that surrounds women's engagement in strength training.

This stigma perhaps lies in a deeply ingrained fear — that by embracing strength training, women risk morphing into caricatures of bulging muscles and hyper-masculine physiques.

However, this apprehension couldn't be further from the truth. Contrary to popular belief, strength training is not a fast track to resembling professional bodybuilders who grace the stage with their sculpted physiques. Achieving such a level of extreme muscularity by professionals requires relentless dedication, rigorous training routines and specialised diets tailored for the competition and usually last only for a short period of time — a path that diverges significantly from the goals of the everyday gym-goer. So unless you are really aiming and training to be a competition-ready bodybuilder, it's impossible to look like one for everyday fitness trainers.

# Finding your gym gear

When it comes to hitting the gym, the question of what to wear can sometimes be as daunting as the workout itself. However, the truth is, there's no one-size-fits-all answer. What you wear should ultimately reflect your personal style, comfort and practicality. Whether you prefer to sport a cute outfit that makes you feel like a fitness goddess or opt for more functional activewear, the key is to find what works best for you.

For those who find motivation in stylish gym attire, there's nothing wrong with a nice outfit that boosts your confidence and gets you excited to break a sweat. Whether it's a matching set of leggings and crop tops or a vibrant tank top paired with colourful shorts, the options are endless. Just make sure that whatever you choose allows for ease of movement and doesn't hinder your workout. On the other hand, if practicality is your main concern, simple and comfortable activewear is the way to go. For women, a pair of leggings or shorts, paired with a supportive gym bra and a top, is all you need to tackle your workout with confidence and for men, a t-shirt with shorts or track pants does the job. Look for fabrics that are breathable, quick-drying and lightweight to help keep you cool and comfortable as you exercise.

When it comes to footwear, the choices can be overwhelming. While there are countless options on the market, finding the right pair for your workout routine is essential. Personally, I've found that shoes with flat soles work best for training. These types of shoes help to keep me grounded on the floor, providing the stability and support needed to lift weights without losing balance. Running shoes, with their curved soles designed for forward motion, may not offer the same level of stability required for training and can sometimes be dangerous, causing you to lose your balance.

I have also seen some gym-goers use Converse Chuck Taylor shoes, known for their flat soles that provide good grip and stability during workouts. Additionally, don't forget about the importance of socks. Opt for sweat-absorbing sports socks to keep your feet dry and comfortable throughout your workout, preventing any slippery sensation between the socks and shoes. I've had great experiences with Lightfeet Evolution socks. While they may lean towards the pricier side, their sweat-proof design makes them a worthy buy. Lightweight and durable, they've served me well over the years, providing comfort and support during countless workouts.

Whatever you wear to the gym should make you feel confident, comfortable and ready to tackle whatever workout lies ahead. The most important thing is to find what works best for you and allows you to perform at your best. So, go ahead, dress for success and conquer your fitness goals with style and confidence.

## Pre-gym consideration

Before you step onto the gym floor, before you grab those weights or hit the treadmill, there's a crucial ritual that can make all the difference between an average workout and a truly exceptional one: pre-gym preparation. It's not just about showing up; it's about ensuring that your body and mind are primed for peak performance.

As we've discussed in earlier chapters, what you eat and how well you sleep directly impact your performance in the gym. The day before your gym session, prioritise nourishing your body with balanced meals and ensuring you get adequate rest and sleep. A meal rich in lean proteins, the right amount of carbohydrates and essential nutrients fuels your muscles and provides the energy needed to power through your workout. If you are into protein shakes, you can also opt to take one right before your workout, which can give you extra energy to power through the workout. Similarly, a restful night's sleep allows your body to be ready for optimal performance.

Why do pre-gym nutrition and sleep matter? Because how you feel on the day of your workout can significantly affect your performance. If you're groggy from a poor night's sleep or sluggish from a heavy, greasy meal, you're more likely to experience fatigue, reduced stamina and diminished focus in the gym. Conversely, when you prioritise your health and well-being and eat clean, you set yourself up for success. But what if you're not feeling your best? What if you're battling a cold or feeling under the weather? In such cases, it's crucial to listen to your body and prioritise your health above all else. Exercising while you are sick can potentially exacerbate your symptoms and prolong your recovery time. Instead, give yourself permission to rest and recuperate and if necessary, seek medical clearance before returning to your workout routine. If you are experiencing symptoms of illness such as fever, body aches, or persistent fatigue, pushing yourself to exercise when your body is already compromised can lead to accidents, injuries and further deterioration of your health.

It's also essential to distinguish between normal tiredness and genuine illness. Feeling a bit fatigued after a long day at work is one thing, but experiencing symptoms of illness is quite another. In the case of normal tiredness, a workout can often provide a much-needed boost of energy and leave you feeling refreshed and invigorated.

## Warm-up exercises

Prepare for success by prioritising the warm-up before hitting the gym. Warm-up exercises prime the body and mind, preparing them for the trials to come. This essential practice isn't merely about physical readiness but also about mental preparation.

By priming the body through dynamic movements, we pave the way for optimal performance while minimising the risk of injury. Each warm-up routine elevates the body temperature and heart rate, facilitating the influx of oxygen to muscles hungry for action. Whether it's a brisk jog on the treadmill, bike, or elliptical or a series of dynamic bodyweight exercises like jumping jacks, arm swings, leg swings, squats and lunges, dedicating just 5 to 10 minutes to warm-up exercises can make all the difference.

# CHAPTER 10:

# THE BASICS OF STRENGTH TRAINING

## Form

My son was one of those babies who struggled to crawl. Instead of using all fours, he dragged his tiny body around the house, relying solely on his right hand. It wasn't until he reached 10 months that he finally figured out the proper form and began to crawl with ease. Once he mastered his true form of crawling, he was able to escape from me at lightning speed whenever I tried to stop him from eating random things. Reflecting on this early experience, I realise the significance of form in every aspect of physical movement. Crawling is the first form of independent human movement that requires patience and practice to master.

Similarly, as we step into the gym, proper form is fundamental to an effective exercise. While there's no shortage of recommended exercises in the fitness world, what often goes overlooked is the education required for executing them in proper form. One session of low weight training with good form is far more effective than countless hours spent in the gym with bad form. So, what exactly is good form? Simply put, it embodies the correct posture and body technique necessary to execute a workout safely and efficiently. It also ensures that we extract the maximum benefit from our workouts, targeting the intended muscles and optimising performance while minimising discomfort and pain.

And what constitutes good form? It begins with standing tall, with the spine straight, head straight and shoulders drawn back. Keeping the neck aligned and the chest lifted fosters optimal breathing and circulation. Meanwhile, maintaining a neutral pelvic position and engaging the abdominal muscles provide stability and support throughout the movements. Softening the knees and elbows prevents locking, safeguarding against strain and potential knee issues.

Mastering proper form does not need to be a daunting task; there are practical strategies to facilitate this process. One effective approach is to practise training in front of a mirror, allowing for real-time feedback on alignment and technique. Recording workout sessions on video can also provide valuable insights into areas for improvement. Alternatively, enlisting the help of a knowledgeable friend or a personal trainer to assess your form and offer guidance can expedite the learning process.

In addition to individual practice, group classes focused on strength training offer a communal environment in which to familiarise oneself with proper form. Led by experienced instructors who demonstrate correct technique, individuals can learn from both the instructor and their peers to gain confidence and competence in refining their form. Some of the bad forms I see regularly at the gym are rounded backs, tensed shoulders, using machines incorrectly, bouncing or swaying while lifting weights, leaning too forward or too backward, ego lifting, and the list goes on.

To maintain good form, start with a comfortable weight that challenges you without sacrificing form or safety. Plant your foot firmly on the ground, maintain balance and use good posture. Breathe properly — exhale as you exert force and inhale while releasing the weights. Steadily concentrate on the muscle you are working on, feeling its engagement with each repetition. And don't rush; avoid ego-lifting beyond your capacity. Remember, you are competing with yourself, not others at the gym. Respect your body's limits and listen to its cues.

For most people, 3 sets of 8 to 12 repetitions with a weight that fatigues the muscles can efficiently build strength and help muscle size. As you get stronger, gradually increase the weight.

A higher number of repetitions with lighter weights will improve muscle tone and endurance, while fewer repetitions with heavier weights will aim to increase muscle size and power. It is essential to structure your training program wisely, ensuring each muscle group is trained 2-3 times per week with adequate rest periods of 1-2 days in between. These intervals of recovery are crucial, allowing muscles to repair and grow stronger. Overtraining should be avoided at all costs, as it can not only hinder progress but also elevate the risk of injury, potentially setting you back as you recover. You don't need to be at the gym every day to see results. Train smarter, not harder, if you want to master fitness and stay fit for life. Overtraining and giving up everything at the gym unless you are training for a competition can lead to burnout and make you more likely to give up too soon. Remember, the key to success is finding a sweet balance between training and enjoying life.

# Mind-muscle connection and muscle activation

The mind-muscle connection is the bridge between intention and action, where the power of our thoughts shapes the outcome of our training. It involves a deliberate act of contracting the muscles while focusing our thoughts on their movement with each repetition, maximising their engagement and potential for growth.

Mindlessly navigating through a workout can prove counterproductive, as less relevant muscles may inadvertently take on more load, leading to imbalances and undesired results. I recall a friend who, despite years of intense leg training, found herself with overdeveloped quads and undertrained glutes. In the end, after years of fitness training, she chose to give up training altogether. To counteract such an imbalance, one must consciously cultivate the mind-muscle connection. Visualisation is a powerful tool in training. By visualising the muscles contracting and relaxing during each repetition, we can enhance their recruitment and activation. Start with lighter weights, allowing yourself to focus on feeling the desired muscles engaged, gradually increasing the weight as your mind-muscle connection strengthens.

Another effective technique is tactile stimulation. By touching and pressing the muscles you wish to engage, you can provide a physical reminder to your body and give them a nudge to wake up for the workout. For instance, I find it harder to feel my shoulder muscles; hence, before my shoulder training, I use a light 1 kg dumbbell to perform a simple single-arm lateral raise and press on my shoulder muscles with my free hand, awakening them from their dormant state. This pre-training activation ensures that my shoulders are primed and ready for the upcoming load. You can apply this same technique to other muscles as well if you want to see them engaged during training.

In my experience, the chest and glutes are the most complained-about dormant muscles in many people. When results are lacking, most people are quick to blame their genetics. The fact is, our bodies are smartly built machines that operate on a "use it or lose it" principle. We sit on our glutes most of the time, leaving these muscles inactive and underutilised. Similarly, our chest muscles often remain dormant because we rely more on our arms and limbs for everyday lifting. Pre-training activation allows the muscles to engage for better results.

By incorporating these techniques into your training regimen, you can harness the power of the mind-muscle connection to unlock new levels of strength and growth, empowering precision and sculpting your physique.

## Progressive overloading

Every morning, my son eagerly joins me in making the bed. It's a simple task, but for him, it's an opportunity to contribute. When he first started walking, he could barely lift the smallest cushion, but with practice, he grew stronger. Slowly but surely, he learned to handle larger pillows until, eventually, he could effortlessly hand me the heavy European cushion, with a bit of exertion and a hint of sweat. This pretty much sums up progressive overloading.

Just as my son gradually increased his ability to handle heavier pillows, progressive overloading involves gradually increasing the intensity and difficulty of your workouts over time. It's about pushing your limits, challenging your muscles and constantly striving for improvement. Imagine performing the same exercises or lifting the same amount of weight day in and day out. While initially effective, this approach eventually loses its potency. The once-challenging weights now feel lighter and the absence of soreness hints at a lack of growth. While reaching a plateau can be a sign of progress in your strength, it also indicates that it's time to shake things up.

Progressive overload is the key to breaking through plateaus and continuing to make gains in your fitness journey. By changing and progressing your workouts, you keep your muscles guessing and force them to adapt and grow stronger. However, it's essential to remember that progressive overload must be approached gradually. Increasing the intensity or frequency of your training too quickly can lead to injury. Just as my son didn't go from lifting small cushions to handling heavy pillows overnight, you shouldn't rush the process of progressive overloading. Instead, approach it with patience and caution and allow up to small increments of weight, up to 10 percent, or add more sets to your sessions.

Incorporating progressive overload into your training regimen can yield remarkable results. It's a simple yet powerful principle that can take your strength level to new heights.

# Consistency

A friend of mine once noticed two gym goers. The first individual, visibly exerting herself with high intensity with messy hair, appeared perpetually exhausted yet failed to reflect the physical transformation. In contrast, the second person oozed an aura of effortless beauty, her commitment seemingly less strenuous yet yielding amazing results. The difference between them is not in effort but in the consistency of their approach. The first individual, perhaps driven by the hope of rapid results, exerted intense effort only to possibly retreat after disappointment. On the other hand, the second individual most likely embraced a steadfast dedication to consistency and discipline, understanding that true progress unfolds gradually over time.

Fitness is indeed a journey — a journey marked by discipline, resilience and trust in the process. It is a journey characterised by the understanding that results are not measured in days or weeks but in months and years. Consistency is not merely about showing up once in a while but about showing up week in and week out, regardless of external circumstances or internal resistance. It is about embracing the process, trusting in the process and making fitness part of your DNA.

Progress is a gradual process that varies from person to person. While some may see progress within months, others may require more time, influenced by factors like body fat composition and their genetics. The crucial element is consistency. Even during weeks when motivation wanes, simply showing up and engaging in minimal training is far better than abandoning the effort altogether. A workout need not be all-or-nothing; even a brief, low-intensity session can keep muscles engaged and the momentum of your progress going. You may think it's only lower intensity, but it still nudges your muscles to stay alert and reminds them that their work is not over yet. Over time, this consistency becomes ingrained, shaping not just your habits but also your very identity.

Despite the temptation to quit when immediate results are not visible, it's vital to remember that muscle growth takes time — typically around 6 to 10 weeks. And if you have fat buildup the muscles won't be visible until there is some fat loss. So, to those who may be disheartened by the absence of immediate results, I offer this simple truth: trust in the process, embrace the journey and remain steadfast in your commitment to your training. In the end, it's not the destination that defines us, but the journey itself.

# CHAPTER 11:

# EXAMPLES OF STRENGTH TRAINING

Welcome to this exciting chapter, where we go through simple workout strategies that you can incorporate into your workout routine. Indeed, the ways in which people approach training vary greatly, influenced by factors such as fitness level, lifestyle and personal preferences. Whether you're a beginner taking your first steps into the world of fitness, an intermediate enthusiast seeking to elevate your workouts, or a seasoned athlete striving for peak performance, the ways in which people train vary significantly.

There is no one-size-fits-all training regimen. The secret to effective training is as much an art as it is a science — a delicate balance of intensity, frequency and variety. There is no hard and fast rule when it comes to crafting the perfect workout plan;

rather, it's about "training smarter". It's about finding what works best for you and your unique circumstances. For the advanced athlete, the focus may lie in muscle isolation training, targeting specific muscle groups with intensity for a sculpted body spread for 5-6 days. However, for most individuals with busy schedules and a desire for overall fitness, simplicity and efficiency are the keys to training smart.

One effective strategy is to incorporate full-body workouts, ensuring that each session engages multiple muscle groups for maximum impact. A personal favourite of mine is the division between upper body and lower body days, which has helped stay fit during postpartum and still have time to enjoy motherhood. It's a balanced approach that allows for comprehensive training without overwhelming complexity. By dedicating separate days to upper and lower body workouts, you engage multiple muscle groups in a single session.

When it comes to structuring workouts, it's essential to consider the unique physiological differences between men and women. Women tend to have proportionally more mass in their abdomen and lower limbs, while men typically carry more mass in their chest and upper limbs. As such, a tailored approach to training frequency and focus is necessary to optimise results. For women, a ratio of 2:1 between lower body and upper body training sessions works well. This means that if you're training three times a week, two of those sessions should focus on the lower body, with the remaining session dedicated to upper body exercises. Additionally, it's important for women to adjust the intensity of their workouts during aunt-flow visitations. Conversely, for men, a ratio of 1:2 typically works well, with one lower body session and two upper body sessions per week.

During my pregnancy, unlike most, I lost a significant amount of weight because I struggled to fit food in my stomach as the baby took up most of the space. On my obstetrician's recommendation, I continued training, but lighter and less frequently. This pregnancy fitness regimen helped me prevent swollen feet and maintain my strength for childbirth. However, my weight ballooned postpartum due to breastfeeding. Despite the massive weight gain, I knew that by staying consistent with my secrets of proper eating and training techniques, I would be okay. A year after my pregnancy, I was back in shape and had no saggy boobs. That was a victory — a victory worth celebrating.

Below are some classic examples of training exercises that you can incorporate into your training sessions. It's important to note that not everyone enjoys the same exercises, so the key is to experiment with various options and pick the ones that you like and enjoy. By finding activities that bring you pleasure and satisfaction, you'll be more likely to stay committed to your fitness routine and achieve long-term success.

# Upper body exercises

A robust upper body is not just for good posture but also essential for functional strength and everyday mobility. Below are examples of various upper body exercises, but not limited to, that effectively target each area:

**Chest:** The chest muscles play a crucial role in pushing movements and stability. Some exercises include the bench press, push-ups, cable chest flys and machine chest press. These movements not only build size and strength but also enhance functional capabilities.

**Back:** A strong back is vital for maintaining good posture, spinal health and overall upper body stability. Exercises such as seated rows, lat pulldowns, bent-over rows, pull-ups and deadlifts target the various muscles of the back. It's also crucial to maintain a balance between chest and back exercises to prevent postural imbalances and reduce the risk of injury. Personally, for me, for every back exercise, I perform an equal amount of chest exercise.

**Shoulders:** The shoulders are a complex joint, comprising several muscles responsible for mobility and stability. Effective shoulder exercises include seated dumbbell shoulder presses, lateral raises, front raises, barbell upright rows, seated machine lateral raises and machine shoulder presses. These movements improve shoulder strength and stability, enhancing performance and reducing the risk of injury during daily activities and sports.

**Biceps and Triceps:** The biceps and triceps are the primary muscles of the arms. Exercises such as hammer curls, concentration curls, barbell curls, preacher-curl machine exercises, seated triceps presses, tricep dips, close-grip bench presses and rope tricep pushdowns target these muscles effectively. Developing strength and definition in the arms enhances functional strength for tasks involving lifting and pushing.

Incorporating a variety of upper body exercises into your workout routine can yield numerous benefits, including improved posture, increased strength, reduced risk of injury and enhanced overall functionality. Whether you're aiming to sculpt a toned physique or simply improve everyday mobility, prioritising upper body training is essential for achieving your fitness goals and maintaining long-term health and wellness.

# Lower body exercises

The lower body comprises some of the largest muscles in the human body, including the glutes and quads. Not only do strong legs provide a solid foundation for movement and balance, but they also play a crucial role in supporting the upper body and enhancing overall fitness. Strong legs are essential for maintaining balance, stability and mobility in everyday activities such as walking, running and climbing stairs. Additionally, the lower body contains the largest muscle mass, making it a prime calorie-burning powerhouse when trained efficiently. By engaging in lower-body exercises, you not only strengthen and tone your muscles but also boost your metabolism and promote overall calorie expenditure for fat loss.

A variety of exercises can target the muscles of the lower body effectively. Squats, lunges, deadlifts, good mornings, leg presses, hack squat machines, leg extensions, seated leg curls and standing calf raise machines are just a few examples of exercises that engage different muscle groups in the lower body. Incorporating a combination of these exercises into your routine can help you develop balanced strength and muscular endurance. It's important not to overload your workout with too many exercises in one session; focusing on 3 to 4 exercises performed effectively is sufficient. Remember, quality prevails over quantity.

# Maximising efficiency with compound exercises

A compound exercise uses multiple muscle groups at once to perform a single movement. By engaging the lower body, upper body and core in one exercise, compound movements offer a comprehensive approach to strength training. Compound exercises offer a time-efficient way to engage multiple muscle groups simultaneously, maximising the effectiveness of your workouts.

By incorporating compound movements like squats, deadlifts, lunges and bench presses, you can engage the lower body, upper body and core in a single exercise, leading to greater calorie burn, an increased heart rate and improved functional strength. For example, a compound deadlift targets not only the glutes and hamstrings but also the quads, forearms, back and abs, making it a highly efficient full-body exercise.

To achieve optimal results from your training, focus on quality over quantity and incorporate compound exercises that target multiple muscle groups. Aim for a balanced workout routine that includes a variety of upper and lower body exercises while allowing for adequate rest and recovery between sessions.

# Cool-down stretches

While the focus of many workouts is on the intensity and duration of the exercise itself, the importance of cooling down should not be overlooked. Just as warming up prepares the body for activity, cooling down is essential for aiding recovery and reducing the risk of injury.

Cooling down serves several crucial functions in the post-workout period. It helps gradually lower the heart rate and body temperature, bringing them back to normal levels. Additionally, cooling down includes stretching exercises that target the muscles trained during the workout. This helps reduce the buildup of lactic acid, which can lead to muscle cramping and stiffness, promoting faster recovery and improved flexibility. Incorporating stretching exercises into your cool-down routine can help alleviate muscle tension and promote relaxation. Here are some effective cool-down stretches to include:

1. **Chest Stretch:** Stand tall with arms extended behind you and interlace your fingers. Gently squeeze your shoulder blades together while lifting your arms, feeling a stretch across the chest.

2. **Hamstring Stretch:** Sit on the floor with one leg extended and the other bent. Lean forward from your hips, reaching towards your toes and feel the stretch along the back of your extended leg.

3. **Back Stretch:** Lie on your back and hug your knees towards your chest, gently rocking side to side to release tension in the lower back.

4. **Foam Roller:** Use a foam roller to massage and release tension in various muscle groups, such as the calves, quads and IT band.

5. **Cobra Pose:** Lie face down with your palms flat on the floor near your shoulders. Press into your hands to lift your chest off the ground, stretching the front of the body.

6. **Child's Pose:** Sit back on your heels with arms extended in front of you and your forehead resting on the mat, feeling a gentle stretch in the back and shoulders.

7. **Overhead Triceps Stretch:** Reach one arm overhead and bend the elbow, placing the hand between the shoulder blades. Use the opposite hand to gently press on the elbow, feeling a stretch along the triceps.

Cooling down after a workout is essential for promoting recovery, reducing muscle tension and enhancing flexibility. By incorporating stretching exercises into your post-workout routine, you can help prevent injury, alleviate muscle soreness and improve overall physical well-being.

# CHAPTER 12:

# HEALING THROUGH FITNESS

In the stillness during my darkest days during the grieving process, when the shattered fragments of my heart seemed irreparable, I found myself staring into the mirror, confronting my inner critic within that echoed my deepest insecurities. "*You are so ugly*", it whispered, "*that your husband doesn't want to be married to you*", so I turned away, avoiding my reflection for days, even weeks, as grief and sadness consumed me.

Lost in my own world of heartbreak, I feared this darkness would swallow me whole, leaving behind nothing but a hollow shell of who I once was. I feared that it was the end for me as the light inside me slowly dimmed. But in the depths of despair, when it felt like the end was near, I found an unexpected lifeline in the strength training. You can't predict what's going to happen to you, but you can change how you react. Feeling drained by the emptiness and hopelessness, I longed to transform my chaotic inner world. Strength training brought mindfulness, where my mind found solace amidst the chaos of my emotions. Fitness taught me to not listen to the unnecessary noises that the mind tells you that "*you are not good enough*" to bring you down, but just be present in the moment and "feel the tension in the muscles". Through mindfulness and self-awareness from training, I learned to silence the cacophony of doubts and fears that once plagued me. I embraced the power of the present moment, finding peace in the simple act of being.

With each lift, each push and each pull, I forged a mind-muscle connection that channelled my pain into purpose. I realised all the pain was helping me evolve into a stronger, wiser version of myself. It was a journey of self-discovery, a path to healing that I hadn't anticipated. My fitness journey was more than just a physical transformation; It was about reclaiming my power and rewriting the narrative of my life. No longer did I see myself through the lens of someone else's rejection; instead, I saw a woman capable of strength and resilience, of overcoming even the darkest period.

As my mindset developed over the years, I watched my body gradually transform, becoming stronger, leaner and more toned.

I also found myself embracing a newfound confidence, not just in how I looked, but in who I was. But it wasn't just about fitting into smaller clothes or achieving a certain look. It was about reclaiming my confidence and learning to love myself exactly as I am.

I remember the first time I looked in the mirror and saw the reflection staring back at me with pride and acceptance. No longer did I shy away from my reflection or criticise not being good enough for someone. Instead, I embraced every curve and imperfection, realising that true beauty comes from within. I began to adorn myself in every outfit, turning even the simplest of garments into a declaration of self-love and acceptance. With each step along this journey, I discovered the beauty of the world anew, its colours more vibrant and its wonders more profound. And as I learned to show kindness and compassion to myself during my training sessions, attuned to my body's cues to push forward or ease back as necessary, I began to extend that same grace to others, becoming more sensitive to the struggles of those around me.

With this newfound confidence came a shift in perspective. As I changed how I viewed myself, I began to see the world in a different light. The colours seemed brighter, the sky seemed bluer, the trees radiated more beauty, smiles felt more genuine and gratitude became endless. But what truly set this transformation apart was that it wasn't just surface level; it came from a place of deep self-love and acceptance. And as I cultivated this sense of awareness and mindfulness, I found myself extending that same kindness and compassion to others.

With this new-found confidence, I ventured to a remote part of Pokhara, located in South Asia, where I volunteered for those who were facing unimaginable hardships. I walked through the hot, rocky roads of the bush and offered assistance in daycares for families struggling to afford childcare who lived on less than a dollar a day. In orphanages filled with children deprived of even the most basic necessities, I witnessed firsthand the stark realities of poverty and deprivation.

Some of the children, whose tiny bodies were ravaged by malnutrition, felt as light as feathers in my arms, which prompted me to discreetly double their lunch portions to ensure they received the nourishment they desperately needed. The satisfaction of secretly aiding these vulnerable children with extra food was unlike any other satisfaction in the world. These childcare facilities were run by charity and their diets consisted only of rice porridge with lentils and a pinch of sugar once a day as a treat. Despite never seeing what lollies or fine food looked like, they remained utterly happy and content.

Despite facing some challenges, such as my clothes getting unintentionally wet as the daycare's children couldn't afford diapers, every moment spent with them filled me with profound joy and sparked a longing desire to experience having a child of my own one day.

With so much to do and so little time, I visited two orphanages and bought them new stationery. I also helped install fans in a boys' orphanage who lived under aluminium-roofed houses where the temperature was so high that one could barely breathe inside. I also had the privilege of speaking with women who had been rescued from human trafficking, offering them a listening ear and words of encouragement. It was a humbling experience, a reminder that our struggles are not isolated, but interconnected, woven into the fabric of humanity.

Despite all the life challenges I faced, including the disappointment of not finding love again, I refused to let my past define me. Instead, I focused on building a future filled with love and purpose. And so, after seven years of healing and growth, I welcomed my baby boy into the world through the gracious gift of a donor, at the age of 41.

The moment I held him in my arms, all the pain and struggles of the past just melted away, replaced by overwhelming joy and gratitude. Becoming a single mother at a later age was not a decision that was made overnight, especially coming from a religious and traditional family and my own personal limiting beliefs, but I knew in my heart it was the right one. It wasn't a decision I made lightly, but rather a profound realisation that my capacity for love was too immense to remain unshared.

I may not have had the traditional family I always dreamed of, but in embracing the unconventional path before me, I discovered a strength I never knew I possessed. Life may not always unfold as we expect, but it is in embracing the journey, with all its twists and turns, that we truly find ourselves.

There were challenges that came from being pregnant and single at an old age. And the challenges came as amplified morning sickness, struggling to do the house chores or missing out on relaxing foot massages, while the struggle of not having a helping hand to tie the shoelaces was painstakingly real. Yet the joy of motherhood, a dream I had eagerly waited for over a decade, seemed to overshadow all these difficulties. I embraced my pregnancy with happiness, proudly carrying my bump and even including it in our family photo with Santa at Christmas time —

just soon to be mom and her baby bump. Each day, I greeted my baby inside my womb with a heartfelt *"good morning"*, *"good night"* and *"I love you"* expressing my love despite not having seen or ever met him. My love for my unborn child filled every moment with joy in my pregnancy journey. Somehow, I felt he knew that he was dearly loved before he was even born.

And just as I gazed at my baby for the first time, a rush of emotions flooded over me. He looked as healthy and vibrant as the walnuts I had diligently consumed throughout my pregnancy — round and plump. His eyes, wide and piercing, seemed to silently convey a profound understanding, as if acknowledging that *"I know that you love me dearly."* Time stood still as I held him close to my chest, every fibre of my being resonating with the realisation that my life had completely changed at that very moment and this time, it was for the better. It was also the moment when I was struck with the realisation: how is it possible that the man I loved so dearly and had known for years brought me so much pain and grief, while a man I didn't even know had given me the most precious gift of my life — my baby boy.

As I navigated the joy and the ups and downs of single motherhood, I realised that none of us have it all together and that's okay. Life can be messy and unpredictable; what we have planned out can be shattered in one moment and the next moment we are completely blessed with life's goodness. Life is beautiful and full of possibility once we open our hearts and minds. And so, I embraced each moment, knowing that every challenge I faced was an opportunity for growth and transformation. In the end, my journey through fitness wasn't just about building a better body; it was about building a better life — one filled with love, acceptance and the courage to embrace whatever comes my way.

And so, as I continue to walk this path of self-discovery and growth, I do so with a heart overflowing with gratitude and a renewed sense of purpose. I know that with each step forward, I am not only transforming my body but also my mind and spirit. And with each triumph, I am reminded of the boundless possibilities that lie ahead, waiting to be embraced with open arms.

# FINAL WORDS

In the labyrinth of our minds, we mostly find ourselves entangled by the web of self-limiting beliefs, those whispered falsehoods that mask as truths, holding us captive in the confines of our own fears. These beliefs, though born from a place of self-preservation, can unwittingly hinder our growth and impede our journey toward self-improvement. Most of the time, we convince ourselves by telling lies such as "I will never overcome my anxiety" or "I am destined to forever struggle with achieving my ideal body weight". But these beliefs are nothing more than illusions, fabrications of our own making of the mind.

The truth is that the power to break free from these self-imposed limitations lies within each and every one of us. It starts with a simple shift in perspective — a willingness to challenge the validity of your beliefs and to recognize that change is not only possible but entirely within your control. Instead of fixating on the enormity of your goals, you can start small, taking gradual steps toward transformation and congratulating yourself on the completion of your small victory. These small steps, one at a time build an unstoppable momentum that creates enormous benefits and results and when you look back and see how far you have come, you will thank those very first few steps.

For instance, set a realistic goal to lose just half a kilo of weight each week and if that seems too big, aim to achieve it in a month or commit to attending just a weekly group fitness class for the first three months to start with. And with each small victory, you can celebrate your accomplishments, acknowledging the strength and determination that reside within you.

As you focus on the three basic pillars of life — eat, sleep and train — you unlock a reservoir of potential, enabling you to sculpt a younger, fitter, happier, stronger and more content version of yourself. Stress acts as a happiness killer and can accelerate the ageing process, but through fitness, we can effectively manage stress. By concentrating on these three fundamental activities, you cultivate a sound mind within a strong body, equipping you to conquer life's obstacles with resilience. With every repetition and every step forward, you edge closer to realising your full capabilities, shedding the layers of uncertainty and self-doubt and helping progress further.

Just as a car requires a balance of brake, clutch and accelerator to navigate smoothly through the roads of life, so too do we require a harmonious blend of eating, sleeping and training to thrive. Sometimes, we must press on the accelerator, pushing ourselves to new heights of physical prowess. Other times, we must ease off the pedal, allowing ourselves the rest and recuperation necessary to heal and rejuvenate. Like a neglected car gathering rust when left idle for too long, our bodies too suffer when we neglect these fundamental pillars of well-being. Even the most sculpted bodybuilder will attest that without consistent care and attention, their physique will wither and fade.

Remember that this is a journey, not a destination. It is an ongoing process — a continuous journey of self-improvement and maintenance. There will be challenges along the way, obstacles to overcome, times when the path may seem too long and moments of doubt that threaten to derail your progress. But through it all, hold on to the belief that within you lies the strength to persevere, to rise above adversity and to emerge with a victory. You have the power inside you to create a better version of yourself. So embrace the journey, celebrate the progress and never underestimate the transformative power that lies within you. You are capable of achieving incredible results. Keep pressing forward, for the best is yet to come.

# THE AUTHOR'S MISSION

In 2019, during a routine health check-up at work, I received unexpected news: my biological age was a staggering 20 years younger than my actual age. The health examiner, baffled by this unexpected result, sought the secrets behind my youthful vitality. Over the past several years, I have amassed a wealth of knowledge in maintaining health and fitness, often fielding inquiries from others who mistook me for someone significantly younger. Whether jokingly attributing it to a mythical fountain of youth or earnestly sharing practical tips, I found joy in helping others in their wellness journeys.

One significant turning point came when I witnessed the transformative impact of health and fitness on my loved ones. Guiding my sister through her post-pregnancy fat loss journey, I witnessed her shed 10 kilograms of body fat in less than a year, thanks to the strategies I shared. Not only did she lose a significant amount of fat, but she also kept it off for the long term. Similarly, when my mother experienced an unfortunate leg fracture and was bound in a foot cast for months, I devised simple yet effective at-home resistance training exercises that helped her regain her strength and muscle mass in her leg after the recovery. Her words of encouragement — that I should consider becoming a personal trainer — ignited a spark of realisation within me. I had the power to effect positive change in people's lives.

Driven by a sense of purpose and a desire to share my knowledge, I pursued and completed Certificate 3 in Fitness. However, I soon realised that my passion lay not in becoming a personal trainer cramped in an hour session but in spreading widely the wisdom accumulated through 27 years of trial and error. Thus, the idea for this book was born — a platform to impart insights on balanced nutrition and effective strength training garnered through years of experimentation.

The truth, as I've come to understand it, is that achieving remarkable results in looking and feeling good is not a privilege only reserved for celebrities and wealthy people. It's a secret accessible to all, irrespective of status or wealth. With this book, I aim to make that journey easier and more accessible for everyone. By offering practical tips on healthy eating and smarter training,

I hope to empower readers to look and feel their best, becoming the best versions of themselves.

If you have been touched and inspired by my stories and tips and are interested in getting in touch, please share your progress and experiences by tagging and posting pictures with #eatsleepandtrain. I would love to see your journey and appreciate your support.

# OPEN LETTER TO MY SON

My dear son, Zion, thank you for being the inspiration for me to write this book. At just over two years old, you are beginning to put words together and my heart warms with joy each time when you call me "*my mama*" and I call you "*my baby*".

Before you were even conceived, I longed for a happy, healthy, loving, intelligent and cute baby. And I have been blessed with just that. Since the moment I discovered I was pregnant, you have brought immense happiness into my life. Becoming a mother was a dream of mine for as long as I can remember and you have gifted me with a motherhood filled with joy and laughter.

I want you to have an abundant life. Spread your wings and embrace all that life has to offer. One day, when you find a beautiful wife, treat her like a queen and shower her with all the love you have to give. Extend the same love and respect to your children and let your love multiply. Raise them with the same love and kindness that I have shown you.

There will be times when you fail. There will be people who judge your choices and tell you that you can't do something or become someone. Do not let others dictate your potential. Never believe that you are not good enough or that you can't achieve your dreams. You "can" do everything that you set your heart and mind to do. You are capable of many great things and all the goodness and abundance life has to offer.

In life, there is power in showing kindness and compassion, even to those who try to bring you down. Everything we experience serves a purpose and it's up to you to navigate the challenges. On days when you feel lost or defeated, look inside your heart and find the strength that lies within. It's the same strength and courage I carried when you were in my womb, telling you every day how you were loved. Be courageous, be bold, live fearlessly and love unapologetically. Do not be afraid to voice your opinions. You are important and your opinions and your thoughts matter. You matter to this world and this world is your oyster.

No matter how the culture tries to portray or belittle women, always respect women. They possess emotional vulnerability yet are capable of nurturing, loving and turning a house into a home filled with care and laughter. The right woman will compliment you, encourage you and stand beside you to help you achieve your goals and visions.

Just as I have filled your cup with love, you have filled my cup overflowingly. I hope one day I can extend my love to those children who are less fortunate than us and be a light in their lives. When you need a listening ear or a shoulder to cry on, trust that I am always here to listen, understand and hug your tears away.

Out of all the women in the world, you chose me to be your mother and for that, I am forever grateful. You have made me the happiest person in the world, and I thank you for choosing me to be your mother.

With all my love,
Mum

# ENDNOTES

1. Some Tips for a good night's rest ...: Melinda Smith, M.A. and Lawrence Robinson, 'How to get a good night's sleep', *How to Sleep Better: Tips to Improve Sleep Quality*, 20 May 2024, www.helpguide.org/articles/sleep/getting-better-sleep.htm

2. The Eat For Health website ...: 'Nutrition Calculators', *Daily nutrient requirements calculator, May 2024*, www.eatforhealth.gov.au/nutrition-calculators/daily-nutrient-requirements-calculator

3. Enjoy a wide variety of nutritious foods from ...: 'Australian Guide to Healthy Eating', *Australian Guide to Healthy Eating*, May 2024, www.eatforhealth.gov.au/guidelines/australian-guide-healthy-eating

4. The recommended protein intake ...: 'Quantity', *How Much Protein Do I Need to Build Muscle?*, June 2024, www.6dsportsnutrition.com/en/science/hoeveel-eiwitten-

nodig-om-spieren-op-te-bouwen#:~:text=The%20 recommended%20amount%20of%20protein,to%2070%20 grams%20per%20day.

5. Healthy oils for cooking ...: 'What does heart healthy eating look like?', *Healthy eating to protect your heart*, June 2024, www.heartfoundation.org.au/healthy-living/healthy-eating/ healthy-eating-to-protect-your-heart

6. Micronutrient deficiencies can cause visible and dangerous health conditions...: 'Micronutrients', *Health Topics*, May 2024, www.who.int/health-topics/micronutrients#tab=tab_1

7. There are several essential micronutrients such as vitamins A, B, C ...: 'Types and functions of micronutrients', *Micronutrients: Types, Functions, Benefits and More*, May 2024, www.healthline. com/nutrition/micronutrients#deficiencies-and-toxicities

8. Free radicals that harm cells, proteins and DNA ...;Jessie Szalay, *'What are Free Radicals'*, June 2024, www.livescience. com/54901-free-radicals.html#:~:text=Oxygen%20in%20 the%20body%20splits,to%20cells%2C%20proteins%20 and%20DNA.

9.  Dietary fibre ...: 'Dietary fibre', *Nutrient Reference Values for Australia and New Zealand, May 2024,* www.eatforhealth.gov.au/nutrient-reference-values/nutrients/dietary-fibre

10. They produce helpful compounds that benefit our overall physical and mental health ...: 'What is gut health and gut microbiome', *Gut health,* May 2024, www.betterhealth.vic.gov.au/health/healthyliving/gut-health

11. The basic tastes, often referred to as ...: Ingrid Appelqvist and Margaret Allman-Farinelli, *'Essentials',* Accounting for taste, *May 2024,* www.science.org.au/curious/people-medicine/accounting-taste#:~:text=Essentials,food's%20smell%2C%20texture%20and%20structure.

12. Some of the benefits of strength training are ...: 'Here are some more benefits of resistance training', 'Benefits of Resistance Training', May 2024, www.revitalizexpp.com.au/benefits-of-resistance-training/

# ABOUT THE AUTHOR

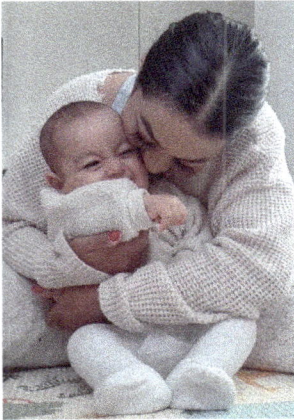

**Diva Selah Joanna** is a devoted mother of one, based in Sydney, Australia. Throughout her life, she has worn many hats. As a young girl, she was a gymnast and loved to sing, and she now thrives in a corporate role as a practising accountant. Her journey as a writer began early, with her first and only article published in her high school magazine, passionately advocating for the revitalisation of a heavily polluted river. This initial foray into writing sparked a lifelong commitment to making a positive impact on the world around her.

Diva's personal story is marked by resilience and determination. Growing up, she faced numerous challenges, including a strict grandfather, her father's failing business, a difficult stepmother, and strained relationships with half-brothers. Despite these hardships, Diva forged a path to success, earning her certification as a practising accountant and securing a stable career in the corporate world. Beyond her professional achievements, Diva is a passionate advocate for personal development, focusing on mental health, strength training, and maintaining a positive outlook on life. She believes in the transformative power of resilience and strength, lessons she has applied in both her personal and professional life.

Diva Selah Joanna is dedicated to inspire and empower others by sharing her journey and insights, offering inspiration and practical advice through her writing. She welcomes feedback and encourages readers to connect with her via email at divaselahjoanna@gmail.com.

www.ingramcontent.com/pod-product-compliance
Lightning Source LLC
Chambersburg PA
CEHW041932260326
41914CB00010B/1266